GOLDENSEAL ROOT:
Your Journey To A Natural Path

By Troy Ellis

Table of Contents

Chapter 1: Goldenseal: A History 1

Use of Goldenseal root in the Native American culture 3

    As an insect-repellent and to treat stomach problems 6

    For clean eyes and disease-free skin......................... 7

    To tackle malaria and other infections 8

Using the Goldenseal root in the modern world 10

Chapter 2: Medical Benefits of Goldenseal 13

The power of berberine and other isoquinoline alkaloids 14

    Berberine to treat cancer patients 17

    Effective in patients suffering from diabetes.......... 20

    Other medical benefits of berberine 21

The many benefits of hydrastine 21

    Antiviral and antibacterial properties 23

    Hydrastine has a significant impact on the uterine muscles 24

    Other use cases of hydrastine 25

Benefits offered by canadine....................................... 27

Another wonder component in the Goldenseal root: Palmatine 31

    Palmatine to treat both neurodegenerative and cardiovascular diseases.. 32

    To treat diabetes and liver-related diseases 35

Other health benefits provided by the Goldenseal root 37

Chapter 3: Goldenseal: An Antibiotic, Antiviral & Antifungal Remedy 41

As a hair tonic for healthier and more luscious hair....43

To deal with bacterial and fungal infections of the scalp 45

Relieving skin conditions like eczema and psoriasis ..46
For better overall digestive health 48
To promote good uterine, urinary, and vaginal health 49
As a natural antiseptic 50
For overall oral health 52
Chapter 4: Rules to Take Goldenseal for Better Health 53
Many forms in which the Goldenseal root is available 53
As raw root 54
As a powder 55
As pills and capsules........................56
As a tincture or extract......................57
In cosmetics and body creams 57
Dosage, frequency, exceptions related to the consumption of the Goldenseal root..........................59
Dosage and frequency 60
Side effects of the rhizome 61
Possible interactions of the Goldenseal root...........63
Usage of the Goldenseal root along with Echinacea 65
Goldenseal root recipes to try out 69
The Goldenseal root infused Tea..........................70
The Elderberry Syrup with Goldenseal and Echinacea...73
The Goldenseal root and Echinacea Jelly...............76
Chapter 5: Conclusion 79
Appendix: References 82

Chapter 1: Goldenseal: A History

Growing mostly in the wild, the Goldenseal is a perennial woodland herb and belongs to the buttercup family Ranunculaceae. Also known as orangeroot, the Goldenseal is native to the eastern United States as well as southeastern Canada. This covers a wide variety of regions, including the northeast border of South Carolina, East to Northern Arkansas, Lower New York, southeast corner of Wisconsin, part of Illinois, as well as Ohio, Kentucky, West Virginia, and Indiana.

The Goldenseal herb produces greenish-white flowers, which later turn into bright red cherries. However, it is not these fruits that make the herb so sought after. Distinguished by its thick yellow root structure, this wonderful herb is characterized by a variety of medical benefits. Native Americans were known to continuously use the Goldenseal root to deal with numerous health ailments. Some of these include:

- Treating skin diseases such as ringworm
- Sore, irritated, and puffy eyes
- As a diuretic drug
- Insect repellent
- Treatment of different types of cancer
- Relieving an upset stomach
- Treating an ulcerated stomach
- Relieve symptoms of jaundice and typhoid fever
- For sore mouths and other gum diseases
- Treating colds and whooping cough
- Treating sore throats
- Treating tonsillitis
- Used as an antiseptic and an astringent
- As an anti hemorrhaging agent
- Treating gonorrhea
- Tending to snake bites

This rhizome is a wonder herb, which, when utilized in a certain form, offers tremendous health benefits. While its medicinal properties were identified and made use of by the Native Americans, Europeans soon began to show considerable interest in the herbal root. After that, commercial pharmaceutical companies began exploring the Goldenseal root as well.

Before we discuss scientifically-backed evidence on the effectiveness of the Goldenseal root for medical ailments and how it can be used safely in the modern world, let us learn about its history in the Native American culture - how and why the Native Americans came to use it.

Use of Goldenseal root in the Native American culture

Wild medicinal herbs have been long used by native cultures all across the world to treat a variety of medical ailments and conditions. The bark of Willow trees was used for headaches, skin sores, fever, and even menstrual cramping. The Cherokees used the Virginia iris to treat several liver ailments. The roots of the wild sage plant were used to help new mothers to recover from childbirth and gain their strength back. Sage was also used for numerous purposes, including bloating, bleeding, bruising, depression, heart diseases, skin diseases, and even excessive sweating.

Witch Hazel was another wild herb that was used by the native tribes to deal with several skin diseases. Smallpox, chickenpox, skin ulcers and sores, and more were treated by using Witch Hazel in different ways. Ginseng was another herb widely used by the Native Americans. Other wild herbs used included sumac, blackberries, rosemary, mint, red clovers, tobacco, sassafras, snakeroot, black gum barks, hummingbird blossoms, wild ginger, lavender, honeysuckle, licorice root, and more. It comes as no surprise that the Native Americans identified Goldenseal in the wild and explored it to be used to treat or relieve symptoms of several diseases.

They found the raw ingestion of Goldenseal to be highly useless. It brought no health benefits to the people. There were negative effects such as burning or tingling feeling, mouth irritation, respiratory issues, and more. In addition, it was also poisonous. Clearly, using it raw and fresh without thorough processing could even lead to death. The Native Americans then realized that to be able to reap the medicinal benefits of the Goldenseal root, they needed to process it first. This would not only remove its poisonous component but also help in broadening its scope of use.

As an insect-repellent and to treat stomach problems

The most popular purpose of the Goldenseal root was to repel insects and avoid any skin diseases or viral infections like the flu, malaria, dengue, and so on. This was incredibly important during the early times since the people didn't have any effective methods of keeping insects away as we do now (mosquito coils and creams). The root of the Goldenseal herb was obtained and left to dry. This dried up rhizome was then converted into a powder. The powder of the Goldenseal root was then mixed with bear fat to prepare a runny mixture. The Native Americans used this mixture to repel insects and keep infections away.

Soon, the Native Americans began to find other purposes for the Goldenseal root as well. An upset stomach was one of their rising concerns. Whether it be diarrhea or an ulcerated stomach, they needed a solution that could work universally. This is where the Goldenseal root turned out to be tremendously useful for them. They either chewed on a clean and fresh root of the Goldenseal herb or a dried-up version of it to relieve stomach concerns. The Goldenseal root also showed healing properties in cases of jaundice. Patients were made to drink a concoction prepared by boiling the Goldenseal root in water.

For clean eyes and disease-free skin

The Native Americans also found the Goldenseal root to be immensely useful in treating a few ailments of the eyes. A wash was prepared using the Goldenseal root to be used to clean out sore eyes and reduce puffiness or inflammation. This was majorly seen amongst the Cherokees of Native America. The Kickapoos of Native America were known for burning the prairies in the autumn after a season of harvest was over. The smoke arising for this huge fire irritated the eyes of many people and caused them to become watery, red, and inflamed. The Kickapoos were able to create a concoction by infusing the Goldenseal root in water. This was then used to treat irritated and sore eyes that resulted from exposure to the smoke.

Goldenseal root was also widely explored and used for its skin-healing properties. Its two most popular forms for this purpose were the wash and the salve. Due to its antiseptic and astringent properties, it was able to treat a variety of issues such as impetigo (which is a contagious skin infection) and ringworm. It has a powerful component named canadine, which acts as a good muscle relaxant.

To tackle malaria and other infections

Goldenseal's powerful deworming and digestive aid properties are attributed to the component called berberine. This component is highly effective in reducing inflammation and treating sores. It acts as an antiseptic against bacteria and protozoa, allowing the patient to recover well without letting the infection spread further. This is why it was also found to be fairly useful in treating pelvic inflammatory disease. Berberine also offers tremendously effective antimalarial properties. It reduces fever in the patient very effectively and prevents the fever from rising back again.

Along with infections of the digestive tract, the Native Americans found the Goldenseal root to be incredibly potent in treating infections of the respiratory mucous tract as well. It also contains two

important components - hydrastine and hydrastine hydrochloride. These are highly effective in treating urinary tract infections and even uterine bleeding. This was widely used in women who went into labor but developed complications during the process. Other than this, the Goldenseal root was also used by the Native Americans as a sedative.

Using the Goldenseal root in the modern world

When the Europeans colonized Native Americans, they diverted their attention heavily towards the medicinal herbs they used. Even though scientific evidence was limited then, the use of numerous herbal medicines, including those made by the Goldenseal root, was very popular. People had hands-on experience in watching someone or themselves recover from ailments by the use of this herb. As the world progressed and modern pharmaceuticals became more prevalent, the use of Goldenseal root became immensely popular as well.

In the early to mid-1800s, commercial production of medicine derived from Goldenseal received a significant boost, and people other than the Native Americans came to use it. The first companies to take an interest in the herb and make it available as tinctures, compounds, dried leaves, dried roots, and powder were Squibb, Parke-Davis, and Lilly, amongst many others. People could now go into health stores all across North America and buy a product of Goldenseal for themselves. Its health benefits were multifaceted, and people were thoroughly impressed by its potency. However, there were rising concerns about its overdosage, which is why modern pharmaceutical companies decided to process the Goldenseal root herb even further.

Parke-Davis, Homeopaths, and Lilly manufactured capsules, oils, tinctures, and tablets that contained the Goldenseal root compound in controlled compositions. This way, people knew exactly how much they should ingest for the required health benefit. Even with its growing popularity and proven positive results, people were still wary concerning its safety. There weren't many scientific studies then to back up the potency of the herb. This did lead to a temporary dip in its usage; however, research and development in the herb brought back the spark in this area. Let us dive deeper into the scientifically-backed information related to the Goldenseal root and how research has been able to solidify its capability in the healthcare industry.

Chapter 2: Medical Benefits of Goldenseal

Goldenseal was originally popularized in the early 1800s by the herbalist Samuel Thompson; however, it still needed scientifically-backed research evidence to gain commercial popularity in the healthcare industry. The threat to its usage by a potential overdose or through side effects (potentially lethal) was too high to be curbed easily by mere claims. People needed solid evidence that the Goldenseal root was safe to use and bore no long-term harmful effects on the human body. A study published in Food and Chemical Toxicology showed that the Goldenseal root was effective in treating infections of the digestive tract, urinary tract, vagina, mouth, and throat. The Goldenseal root not only helps in dealing with a wide variety of ailments but also has a powerful potential to stop cancerous growth in the human body. Let us dig deeper into the scientific reasoning behind why the Goldenseal root carries such powerful medicinal and healing properties.

The power of berberine and other isoquinoline alkaloids

Research found that the Goldenseal root contains isoquinoline alkaloids that carry tremendous health benefits. While these isoquinoline alkaloids as a solvent or a corrosion inhibitor, their antimicrobial, antiseptic, astringent, and anti-inflammatory properties have helped treat a wide variety of medical ailments. One of the most important chemicals found in Goldenseal root is berberine. It is also found in other wild herbs, including European barberry, Oregon grape, tree turmeric, and goldthread. It is also this berberine that gives the Goldenseal rhizome its unique golden color.

The most distinctive property of berberine is its antimalarial properties. It is a powerful agent to help reduce fever and treat the infection that's causing it as well. It is also a powerful contender to treat inflammation and sores because of its antibacterial properties. A study published in Oxford Academic and the National Library of Medicine showed the positive effects of berberine in treating cutaneous leishmaniasis using high doses over ten days. (Cutaneous leishmaniasis is a skin disease that causes an infection due to the bite of a parasite. It is a very common disease affecting humans and is most commonly found in tropical and subtropical areas.)

The Goldenseal root was traditionally and historically immensely popular in dealing with issues related to the eyes. Whether it was inflamed and watery eyes or irritated eyes, the Goldenseal root always proved beneficial in relieving the symptoms and treating the issue well. Berberine has proven to be exceptionally capable of treating eye-related inflammation and irritation. A study published in the Journal of Clinical Therapeutic showed that berberine is a therapeutic alkaloid exceptionally useful in treating clinically positive trachoma patients. Berberine was shown to significantly reduce inflammation and provide tremendous relief to the patients.

Another powerful use of the isoquinoline alkaloids in the Goldenseal root is in treating medical conditions of the stomach - ulcerations in the stomach, an upset stomach, infections of the stomach and digestive tract, worms in the stomach, and more. Its antimicrobial and deworming properties make it possible to deal with such stomach and digestive tract related issues effectively. A study published in the National Library of Science talks about how berberine has growth-inhibiting effects on human intestinal bacteria, thereby relieving symptoms of stomach infection and deworming the stomach of any microbes. Another study published in Indian Pediatrics has proven the positive effects of berberine in treating diarrhea.

These, in turn, are great properties to deal with illnesses of the liver and kidney as well. It helps bring down the high levels of cholesterol and other lipids in the body as well as lowers the blood pressure. It shows great capability in dealing with typhoid fever and treating its symptoms completely. Berberine is also a good diuretic agent. This means that liver and kidney patients who suffer from the improper discharge of body fluids can benefit from the usage of Goldenseal root. It promotes diuresis, which causes you to excrete toxic waste via your urine.

Berberine to treat cancer patients

There is no cure for cancer yet. Current treatment options are mostly limited to radiation therapy and chemotherapy drugs. While these are beneficial in some patients, others are resistant. There is no guarantee of whether cancer would go away permanently or not. Numerous other alternative medicines (CBD drugs, liposomal CBD) are now being used to at least relieve some of the symptoms. Any safe and viable treatment option in this respect has always been welcomed. Goldenseal root is a promising candidate in this matter, and its potency has also been supported by a wide variety of scientific research. However, to be used as a mainstream method of treatment, there is still a long way to go for this isoquinoline alkaloid.

A study published in the Journal of Ethnopharmacology proved that berberine was a powerful isoquinoline alkaloid agent to prevent the growth of cancer cells in the human colon. The cyclooxygenase-2 transcriptional activity is an important step in the tumor to replicate its DNA and form new cancer cells. If this process is completed successfully, the cancer cells grow in number and size and makes the cancerous tumor worse. However, the inhibition of this activity would cause the tumor cells to prevent any transcription and thus stop its growth immediately. This study was able to prove that berberine has inhibitory properties that bring the cyclooxygenase-2 transcriptional activity to a complete stop.

Another research was carried out by a team of researchers and was published in the Cancer Letters journal in January 2000. Esophageal cancer cells were taken in vitro and treated with an abundant dose of berberine. It was found that the berberine had a powerful inhibitory effect on the cancer cells and restricted their growth in the esophageal tract completely. Another study published in the International Journal of Experimental and Clinical Pathophysiology and Drug Research found that berberine again had inhibitory effects on the cyclooxygenase-2 transcriptional activity in oral cancer cells. These studies have tremendously solidified the position of Goldenseal root to be used as an alternative medicine to treat cancer.

Effective in patients suffering from diabetes

Diabetes is an incredibly uncomfortable and stressful medical condition to live with. You cannot have any sugary food items, you tend to urinate more often, your blood pressure is always off the charts, and you regularly feel tired and out of breath. These are just a few symptoms of diabetes. With age and intensity of diabetes, the condition worsens further. The berberine chemical in the Goldenseal root has been found to be thoroughly effective in dealing with symptoms of diabetes. A semi-high dose of berberine (prescribed by a doctor) can help reduce blood sugar levels effectively.

A study published in the Chinese Journal of Modern Developments in Traditional Medicine proved the therapeutic effect of berberine in 60 patients who were suffering from Type II Diabetes Mellitus. Another study conducted by the Department of Chemistry and Biochemistry, Calvin College, Grand Rapids, proved that berberine showed hypoglycemic effects (reduction in blood sugar levels). This effect was shown by berberine and was attributed to the acute activation of the transport activity of GLUT1. Clearly, berberine is a powerful contender of alternative medicine to treat diabetes patients.

Other medical benefits of berberine

Another health benefit of berberine is in the treatment of heart-related medical problems. Several scientific research has shown that berberine is successful in reducing the levels of total cholesterol by 24 mg/dL, LDL cholesterol by 25 mg/dL, and triglyceride levels by 44 mg/dL. A study published in the Clinical Cardiology journal showed that berberine was able to effectively treat patients suffering from severe congestive heart failure. Moreover, diabetes and high blood pressure are severe risk factors that increase the severity of heart diseases. Since berberine is effective in reducing the severity of these conditions as well, it is highly useful in dealing with heart-related problems.

Sepsis is another medical condition that berberine has been found to be useful for. It results from a massive immune response to a bacterial infection. The antimicrobial properties of berberine are highly effective in dealing with this condition. The antimicrobial and fever-reducing properties of berberine also makes the Goldenseal root a perfect treatment method against pneumonia. This isoquinoline alkaloid has also been found to be incredibly effective in dealing with PCOS (Polycystic Ovarian Syndrome) in women. A person suffering from PCOS usually suffers from high blood pressure and cholesterol, as well as high severity of diabetes. Since berberine has been useful in treating these symptoms, it is also effective in reducing the severity of PCOS.

These are mostly health benefits of the isoquinoline alkaloid, berberine. However, berberine isn't the only isoquinoline alkaloid found in the Goldenseal root. Hydrastine, canadine, and hydrastine hydrochloride are other isoquinoline alkaloids found in the Goldenseal root. These isoquinoline alkaloids offer additional medical benefits ranging from treating uterine bleeding, acting as a muscle relaxant, dealing with infections and inflammations, and also being used as a sedative. Let us have a closer look at the scientific studies conducted in this aspect and how these isoquinoline alkaloids help treat and manage various health conditions.

The many benefits of hydrastine

There's no doubt that one single chemical cannot be the hero of any wild medicinal herb. Numerous such components come into play to make the herb a powerful remedy against various medical problems, and this is where another isoquinoline alkaloid, hydrastine, has shown tremendous capability. Hydrastine undergoes a reaction called hydrolysis (a chemical reaction where a substance breaks down due to its interaction with water). Upon hydrolysis, hydrastine produces hydrastinine, which is a hemostatic drug. A hemostatic drug helps in dealing with accidental blood flow. The discovery of this alkaloid in 1851 by Alfred P. Durand was a revolutionary step in medical science and healthcare.

While the human body requires a continuous and steady flow of blood to maintain healthy body functions, sometimes, the prevention of blood flow becomes necessary. One might suffer from a brain hemorrhage (which refers to the loss of blood by the organ, often as internal bleeding) and require medical intervention from preventing the blood from pooling in the head and resulting in multiple organ failure. There are also some people who are not able to heal their internal wounds quickly and thus need something to speed up the process for them so that they do not lose any more blood. Prevention of blood flow might also be needed in pregnant women who have gone into labor and become subject to uterine bleeding during the process.

For all such cases, it is crucial to provide medical intervention as soon as possible and prevent the flow of blood immediately to ensure that the patient doesn't undergo multiple organ failure. Hydrastine plays an important role in helping healthcare professionals achieve this. Hydrastine quickly undergoes hydrolysis and produces hydrastinine, which is an effective agent to stop the flow of blood. When given in the right dosage and at an appropriate time, hydrastine can save lives very easily. This spectacular property of hydrastine, found in the Goldenseal root, made the herb an exceptionally rare find.

Antiviral and antibacterial properties

Berberine offers numerous antimicrobial properties that make it a great candidate to fight against infections or viral fever. However, the power of the Goldenseal root in dealing with such medical conditions isn't limited to the presence of berberine alone. According to an academic paper by the University of Colorado, hydrastine was found to possess remarkable antibacterial and antiviral properties. Hydrastine and berberine combined serve as an exceptional agent to deal with any bacterial or viral infections such as strep throat, urinary tract infections, food poisoning, gonorrhea, chlamydia, syphilis, the flu, and even chickenpox. Since berberine is also a great candidate to be used against skin infections, combining it with hydrastine offers an additional layer of treatment against bacterial skin infections.

Hydrastine has a significant impact on the uterine muscles

The Native Americans were known for using the Goldenseal root to help menstruating women or women in labor. They often used the Goldenseal root to induce labor in a pregnant woman who had significantly crossed her gestation period. The Goldenseal root was also used in higher quantities to relax the uterine muscles in other cases. While the first known use of commercial Goldenseal root manufactured by pharmaceuticals rarely included uterine problems, further scientific research provided a lot of solid evidence to support this. In these lab studies, it was found that hydrastine shows considerably positive results when used to stimulate the uterine muscles.

Hydrastine is a powerful agent to be used to induce contractions even today. If approved by your doctor, you can use the Goldenseal root to make use of the properties of hydrastine to bring about this effect. In some serious cases of labor, women even begin to bleed vaginally. There are also chances that the lives of both the mother and the baby are in danger. If this is allowed to continue, the patient can lose a significant amount of blood from their bodies. Since hydrastine is a hemostatic drug and is present in high quantities in the Goldenseal root, it can be used to stop these uterine bleedings and save the patient's life.

Other use cases of hydrastine

A study published in the National Library of Science states that the Goldenseal root was phenomenally useful and effective in bringing the chronic inflammation in the lungs and the nasal tract to a significant minimum. Hydrastine, coupled with the benefits of berberine, offers an exceptionally good digestive environment. This rhizome is a powerful agent to treat ailments of the digestive tract and promote defense against harmful microorganisms. Hydrastine works to significantly increase the production of immunoglobulin. This is an important chemical required to boost your intestines' strength against infections. With levels of immunoglobulin increased, you can prepare yourself against any such ailments.

Additionally, hydrastine is also a very good agent to deal with skin infections. Since it offers numerous antimicrobial, anti-inflammatory, and antiseptic properties, a wide variety of skin infections can be treated using commercially manufactured products of the Goldenseal root. Plus, it adds to the power of berberine in dealing with such issues as well. In severe lab cases of acne, a patient was put on high doses of commercially derived hydrastine extract. Acne is caused when the bacteria, Propionibacterium acnes, sits on your vulnerable skin and infects it. The result is an inflamed, irritated, infected, and patchy skin. In a matter of six weeks, the patient was completely cured, and signs of improvement could be seen as early as ten days.

Other than severe cases of acne, hydrastine is also a good alternative medicine to deal with eczema of the face, anus, ears, feet, and scalp. It is also useful in people who grow beards and often suffer from inflamed hair follicles. Usage of hydrastine in such cases not only reduces inflammation but also helps in treating any bacterial infections. Mild to high dosage of hydrastine is also very beneficial in dealing with excessive sweating. People who suffer from excessive sweating, especially under their arms, do not find many solutions to deal with the situation. Using an aqueous solution of the Goldenseal root can be very useful in such cases.

Benefits offered by canadine

The third most important isoquinoline alkaloid present in the Goldenseal root is canadine. Although not many commercially available variants of the Goldenseal root have canadine as a major constituent, this isoquinoline alkaloid is still crucially important. However, the limited knowledge that we have on canadine can easily be attributed to the fact that a lot of research and development is carried out in hydrastine and berberine. Since these two isoquinoline alkaloids are present in high quantities and provide treatment options and defense against a wide variety of medical ailments, a lot of focus is given to them. The idea is to obtain more solid evidence for both of these isoquinoline alkaloids and ensure that no stones are left unturned in exploring their powerful capability.

A few of the research studies carried out by keeping canadine in focus have found out that canadine offers phenomenal antioxidative properties. A 2008 study published in the Bioorganic and Medicinal Chemistry journal found out that the stereoelectronic properties of canadine are very similar to alpha-tocopherol. These similarities point towards a powerful antioxidative nature of canadine. Continued research in this domain can help the Goldenseal root to become a mainstream antioxidant agent in the pharmaceutical market. This study also found that unlike other trace isoquinoline alkaloids found in the Goldenseal root - anonaine and antioquine - canadine possesses no cytotoxic effects. This means that its use in the human body for medicinal purposes would not pose any threat to the living cells. This is a strong point for the Goldenseal root to establish itself as a commercial alternative medicine used widely by the healthcare industry since it would not cause any threat to human life.

Apart from this antioxidant and non-cytotoxic nature, canadine also promotes myogenesis. Myogenesis refers to the formation of muscular tissue. This process is exceptionally important in human beings, especially in the embryonic stages of development. Any hindrances in this process can cause your muscles to become weak and your movements to be uncoordinated. Furthermore, it can get very difficult to move around in the later stages of life. It was found that canadine doesn't just promote the process of myogenesis but also prevents muscle protein from degradation. This makes it a strong muscle growth agent to be used in patients who are suffering from degenerating muscle tissues.

Because of this property, canadine can also be used as a muscle relaxant. The Native Americans widely used the Goldenseal root to relax muscles in cases of a sprain or muscle injury. It was because of canadine that the Goldenseal root was used to deal with strained muscles. They usually prepared a salve or a rub out of the Goldenseal root and used it for this purpose. In some cases, the Goldenseal root was also boiled in water, and the concoction thus prepared was drunk to relieve muscles. Other than these, canadine is also a good sedative. It can induce a calm and relaxing sleep and can be very useful to help patients suffering from depression, anxiety, or insomnia.

Another wonder component in the Goldenseal root: Palmatine

Whenever it comes to discussing the Goldenseal root and its medical benefits, a lot of attention is often garnered by its major isoquinoline alkaloid, berberine. Berberine is also the one regarding which abundant research has been carried out. Most commercially available Goldenseal root products also contain berberine as a major constituent. Other chemicals to gain more attention are hydrastine and canadine. However, there are still not many commercially available pharmaceutical products that have hydrastine and canadine in abundance. This changed when significant research was done to find the medical benefits of another isoquinoline alkaloid present in the Goldenseal root - Palmatine.

In a review included in the Phytotherapy Research journal, it was found that palmatine not only helps to deal with medical ailments like inflammation, hypertension, and dysentery but also liver-related problems such as jaundice. Its anti-inflammatory properties make it possible for it to be used in even severe cases of inflammation. This level of potency hasn't been shown by any isoquinoline alkaloid present in the Goldenseal root other than berberine. In fact, the health benefits offered by palmatine might even surpass those offered by berberine. It won't be long before more commercially produced Goldenseal products have palmatine as the major constituent and not berberine. This is attributed to the fact that numerous studies are finding out several medical benefits of palmatine.

Palmatine to treat both neurodegenerative and cardiovascular diseases

One of the most exciting discoveries about palmatine is that it has a positively enhancing effect on the Nerve Growth Factor or NGF. The Nerve Growth Factor is associated with neurons in the human brain. A high level of this Nerve Growth Factor indicates that the growth, maintenance, and survival of specific neurons are being carried out effectively by the human body. Nerve Growth Factor is an important factor in play when it comes to determining the health of a person's brain. A low level of Nerve Growth Factor indicates that the person's neurons aren't growing or surviving well. Such degenerating neurons can directly lead to numerous neurodegenerative diseases, including Alzheimer's disease, Parkinson's, Schizophrenia, and other types of Dementias. Other medical conditions arising from a low level of the Nerve Growth Factor also include Rett Syndrome, bipolar disorder, and autism.

Additionally, the Nerve Growth Factor also contributes to several medical conditions not related to neurons directly. Low levels of Nerve Growth Factor contribute to cardiovascular diseases such as atherosclerosis, diabetes, and obesity. The levels of the Nerve Growth Factor can be improved in
the human body with the intake of the Goldenseal root. The palmatine in this wild herb helps tremendously with maintaining healthy levels of the Nerve Growth Factor. Recent studies have found that by increasing the output of

neurite, palmatine is able to give the Nerve Growth Factor a significant boost. It's interesting to note here that berberine also shows these attributes; however, palmatine has been found to be more effective in doing so.

Thus, palmatine can be highly beneficial in treating a range of neurodegenerative diseases and keeping their symptoms at bay. Overall, if a patient suffering from a neurodegenerative disease is put on a dosage of any product derived from the Goldenseal root, they might be able to receive all-round medical care. Berberine can help reduce the inflammation in brain tissues, canadine can offer relief from depression and violent episodes by working as a sedative, and palmatine can help reduce the intensity of the neurodegenerative disease by increasing the levels of the Nerve Growth Factor to optimum levels.

It can also help in reducing the intensity of cardiovascular diseases and treating them completely. A study published in the journal of the Federation of American Societies for Experimental Biology found that palmatine was able to show positive effects in treating cardiovascular diseases and also offered low toxicity. Additionally, palmatine also possesses antidiabetic properties, which can thus help in treating Type II Diabetes Mellitus. Thus, not only can medically-approved doses of the Goldenseal root provide great relief from neurodegenerative diseases but also offer a good alternative medicine candidate to deal with chronic cardiovascular conditions such as severe atherosclerosis.

To treat diabetes and liver-related diseases

A study published in October 2015 talks about how palmatine can be a very effective agent to treat diabetes. Diabetes Mellitus is characterized by hyperglycemia, which means that a person's blood sugar levels reach levels that are higher than the appropriate mark. To be able to deal with diabetes, a person needs to take proactive steps towards keeping their blood sugar levels in check and ensuring that they take appropriate measures in the case that it does go beyond the optimum levels. This is where the isoquinoline alkaloid, palmatine, present in the Goldenseal root comes into play. The study showed that palmatine was highly effective in reducing plasma blood sugar levels in the rat model.

The positive control in this study was kept as Tolbutamide. This is a synthetic compound that is used in the treatment of diabetes patients very commonly. Tolbutamide is one of the most effective agents in reducing blood plasma sugar levels. In this study, the researchers found that not only was palmatine effective in bringing a significant decrease in blood plasma sugar levels, but it was able to do so much better than Tolbutamide. It also reduced the oxidative stress levels in the rat model, which is highly important for patients suffering from diabetes. This study clearly proves that the palmatine chemical present in the Goldenseal root can be very effective in managing diabetes in human patients as well.

Apart from this, palmatine is also an effective agent to deal with liver-related issues. Jaundice is one of the most common conditions related to the liver. Bilirubin is a yellowish bile pigment secreted by the liver to carry out effective biochemical reactions that assist in sustaining the human body. When the liver begins to secrete this bile pigment in very high quantities, the human skin begins to turn yellow. It can also occur if your liver fails to produce red blood cells effectively. Studies have shown that palmatine is a very good agent to try and treat this medical condition.

Other health benefits provided by the Goldenseal root

The above-mentioned health benefits of the Goldenseal root have been strongly supported by numerous scientific studies. These studies have also given a push to the commercial production of Goldenseal products by numerous pharmaceutical companies all across the world. However, it is very interesting to note here that these aren't the only medical conditions that the wonderful yellow rhizome can treat. Even though the evidence related to these other health benefits is limited, there are a few studies that point out the untapped potential of this wild herb. While we wait on receiving further insights on these added health benefits, it is still crucial to discuss the possibility of more problems being solved.

One of the most important medical benefits that the Goldenseal root might provide is related to your oral health. There is evidence, even though limited, that Goldenseal is a great agent to treat tooth infections. The Native Americans were rumored to use the Goldenseal root to treat their gum problems; however, there wasn't a lot of scientific backing to this claim. A study published in the Journal of Clinical and Diagnostic Research found out that the isoquinoline alkaloids present in the Goldenseal root are highly effective in reducing the growth of bad bacteria in our mouth. This helps with keeping oral diseases such as gingivitis and dental plaque at bay. Another study published in the International Dental Journal states that a solution form or paste form of processed Goldenseal root is a great substance to be used as either mouthwash or toothpaste. It not only kills bacteria but also helps with relieving inflamed gums.

While the Goldenseal root has been clinically effective in treating numerous skin conditions such as infections, eczema, acne, and skin inflammation, new evidence suggests that it might also be useful in dealing with psoriasis. In psoriasis, the patient's skin cells multiply at a rate of ten times the usual and form bumpy, red, and inflamed patches all over the body. It is a highly uncomfortable skin condition where medical intervention is required without fail. Not many treatment options are available for this condition, and ointments or light therapy can only offer a little relief. A recent 2017 study found out that the Goldenseal root possesses antipsoriatic and anti-inflammatory properties strong enough to treat psoriasis effectively.

Last but not least, the Goldenseal root could also be used as a mainstream drug to treat a variety of sexually transmitted diseases or STDs (HIV, Hepatitis, Chlamydia, Herpes, Syphilis, and others). Even though the positive effects of hydrastine have been established in this matter, researchers are still not sure about the toxicity that these chemicals can pose to humans. This is why further research is required in this matter. However, a few select studies claimed that when the preparation of the Goldenseal root was mixed with thyme and myrrh, it was found to be effective in reducing the symptoms of and treating oral herpes.

Chapter 3: Goldenseal: An Antibiotic, Antiviral & Antifungal Remedy

Till now, we have mostly talked about the properties of Goldenseal as a medicinal agent for when we fall ill. Whether it is a neurodegenerative disease like Alzheimer's or irritated eyes or even a skin condition like ringworm, the Goldenseal root has proven to be immensely effective. With continued research in the goodness of this yellow rhizome, it is expected to become a mainstream alternative form of medicine to treat several diseases. Soon, healthcare professionals will be able to prescribe products and drugs derived from the Goldenseal root as a standalone medicine. However, this is not the only way the Goldenseal root has proven itself to be useful.

The Goldenseal root has powerful antibiotic, antiviral, and antifungal properties. The isoquinoline alkaloids - especially berberine, hydrastine, and palmatine - are immensely powerful in dealing with a wide variety of problems.

However, these isoquinoline alkaloids also come with very low toxicity. This means that not only can they be used to treat medical conditions but can also be utilized as an everyday remedy for the overall wellbeing of the human body. This is where one of the most powerful capabilities of the Goldenseal root comes into play. Because of its great antibiotic, antiviral, and antifungal health benefits, the Goldenseal root is an amazing everyday herb.

The isoquinoline alkaloids is not the only thing that makes the Goldenseal root so powerful; it's also rich in vitamins A, B, C, and E. In addition, it houses an abundance of minerals such as potassium, calcium, iron, and zinc, amongst many others. Other than these, the Goldenseal root also has good fatty acids that assist in carrying out crucial biochemical functions in the human body.

Clearly, the Goldenseal root is a powerhouse of essential chemicals that helps one become immensely healthy. Therefore, its consumption helps raise your immune system, thus keeping diseases at bay. Let us have a closer look at how you can use the Goldenseal root as a wonder herb for your everyday woes.

As a hair tonic for healthier and more luscious hair

Your hair needs a host of vitamins and minerals to grow healthy and luscious. Not taking proper care of your hair would cause them to become dull, dry, and lose all their shine. In today's world, where pollution is rampant, and the exposure to the sun is at an all-time high, we need something more than just shampooing and oiling the hair to help them stay shiny and healthy. Vitamin A is essential to induce hair growth and keep the scalp moisturized (not oily). Vitamin B helps carry essential nutrients to the hair follicles to keep them strong and smooth. There's also Vitamin C that produces collagen - the structural foundation of hair. So, your hair needs to keep oxidative stress at bay to ensure that they are healthy. This is where Vitamin E comes into play.

Other than these vitamins, your hair also needs a lot of iron and zinc. Iron helps carry oxygen to your hair follicles to keep them strong. It also prevents a condition called anemia, which is the leading cause of hair fall. On the other hand, zinc helps in hair tissue growth as well as repair of damaged hair follicles. This is essential to keep dry and split ends at bay. Now, bringing all of these benefits together in one single pill or herb is not easy. However, this is where the Goldenseal root can help. Since it is rich in Vitamins A, B, C, and E and also has iron and zinc in abundances, it can be used as an effective hair tonic for healthier and more luscious hair.

One can use the Goldenseal root to protect their hair from the pollution outside, sun exposure, and even our poor dietary habits. Modern pharmaceutical companies offer Goldenseal root products in various forms. To derive its benefits for your hair, one of the best ways to consume the Goldenseal root is in its powder form. For those who are not comfortable consuming the powder or find it difficult, the Goldenseal root products can also be used as a liquid concoction. Applying the liquid form of the Goldenseal root directly on your hair can be immensely beneficial for their health and growth as well.

To deal with bacterial and fungal infections of the scalp

Your hair's growth and health is also affected by bacterial and fungal infections of the scalp. An unhealthy scalp can severely impact your hair's growth. Hence, an infection of the scalp can also be highly uncomfortable and irritable. Increased inflammation of the scalp can even lead to cracking of the skin and bleeding. One of the most common fungal infections of the scalp is dandruff. In mild cases, dandruff can be easily treated with an anti-dandruff shampoo. One can even use a lemon solution to deal with the issue. However, severe cases of scalp infection need more attention than just that. The Goldenseal root possesses brilliant anti-inflammatory and antimicrobial properties owing to the powerful isoquinoline alkaloid, berberine. When you use any form of the Goldenseal root to deal with bacterial or fungal infections of the scalp, you can see improvements within a week. The redness and itching on the scalp due to the infection will reduce significantly. You will also begin to see a lot of improvement in the symptoms of the infection itself. The dry flakiness begins to reduce, and your scalp begins to get better slowly and steadily. The good thing about the Goldenseal root is that it can be used regularly as well. You can continue to use it for healthy and luscious hair while also keeping any scalp infections away.

Relieving skin conditions like eczema and psoriasis

Skin infections like eczema and psoriasis cannot be treated in the short-term. It takes a long time to relieve its symptoms. Additionally, there are several cases where these conditions are not treated completely as well. Now, since the treatment methods of these skin conditions require long-term care, the Goldenseal root is a great candidate to be used as an alternative medicine to deal with these conditions. The Goldenseal root products reduce the inflammation and the flakiness of the skin condition. It also helps the skin in defending itself against the microbes and promoting healthier skin.

Using the Goldenseal root regularly can also help to prevent these problems. It promotes an overall healthy skin and helps you keep harmful microbes away. It also helps prevent fungal skin infections such as ringworm or athlete's foot. The Goldenseal root has powerful antiseptic and astringent properties. This means that using it as an everyday herb would prevent such fungal infections from happening in the first place. Moreover, the Goldenseal root can also be used to deal with blisters and sores. Whether they arise from harsh sun exposure or due to an accidental infection, the isoquinoline alkaloids are highly effective in dealing with blisters and sores and treating the problem at the grassroot level.

For better overall digestive health

Berberine is an important isoquinoline alkaloid present in the Goldenseal root. It is also the primary component in a majority of the commercially produced Goldenseal products. Berberine is a powerful agent for good digestive health. It helps with tackling bad bacteria in the digestive system and keeps indigestion away. The Goldenseal root is also effective in treating stomach or intestinal infections such as food poisoning, intestinal infections, and so on. It gives a good boost to digestive enzymes, thus making sure that no interruptions are faced in the entire digestive tract. Moreover, the Goldenseal root is also very effective in stimulating hunger in our bodies.

This is very useful in treating patients who are suffering from anorexia. It stimulates hunger and helps people better their eating habits. This is also very effective in patients who are suffering from depression and anxiety. A person suffering from clinical depression or anxiety usually deals with a host of other symptoms. One such symptom is the loss of appetite. In many severe cases, patients have difficulty keeping their food down. This aversion to food causes the patients to become incredibly weak and tired as well. The Goldenseal root is a good alternative medicine to deal with this issue. It helps the patient to start wanting to eat food and developing a healthy appetite.

To promote good uterine, urinary, and vaginal health

The isoquinoline alkaloids in the Goldenseal root help women deal with a variety of vaginal, urinary, and uterine problems. One of the most common problems suffered by a woman is urinary tract infection. It can be contracted very easily and causes a lot of discomforts such as painful urination, inflammation of the urinary tract, and more. The anti-inflammatory and antimicrobial properties present in the Goldenseal root help tackle urinary tract infections effectively. The antimicrobial properties help with tackling the infection and relieving symptoms of the infection. Plus, the anti-inflammatory properties help with dealing with the inflammation, pain, and discomfort while urinating.

Another common medical problem associated with women's reproductive health is menstrual cramps. While some people do not experience a lot of menstrual cramps, many find it incredibly painful. Products made from the Goldenseal root can help with relieving menstrual cramps. The isoquinoline alkaloids present in this are very effective in relieving contractions of the uterine muscles and dealing with the pain. Consumption of the Goldenseal root regularly can help women deal with such uterine, urinary, and vaginal problems and promote overall good health of their bodies.

As a natural antiseptic

Getting snips and cuts on your fingers, arms, or legs is very common. Your cuts can be large from a fall or a simple knife cut when cutting vegetables or fruits. Most small cuts heal on their own, but larger cuts require medical attention. Some small cuts may need medical care if they have been from a dirty surface. For example, if you get a small cut from a dirty iron piece, you need to get medical attention right away. These small cuts can get badly infected and turn gangrene as well. This is why it is crucial to use an antiseptic and clean out the wounds immediately. You also need an antimicrobial to kill any bad microbes that might have gotten into the cut.

While there are numerous antiseptics and antimicrobials in the pharmaceutical market, one of the most effective and useful ones is the products derived from the Goldenseal root. They are available as aqueous solutions and can be used as a powerful antiseptic and antimicrobial. The isoquinoline alkaloids, especially berberine, are very capable of killing the microbes and cleaning out the cuts. Since it also has anti-inflammatory properties, if any of these cuts result in inflammation or severe pain, the Goldenseal root products can help bring down that inflammation as well. Thus, keeping a Goldenseal root product in your first aid kit and using it as a natural antiseptic is always a good idea!

For overall oral health

Oral health is an everyday struggle, and it takes a lot to manage it well. Brushing your teeth regularly and with good toothpaste is crucially important. Not doing so can result in a lot of dental problems. Gingivitis, dental plaque, sore and bleeding gums, and more are very common oral problems and need a lot of attention to treat these conditions completely. The Goldenseal root is crucially effective in dealing with these dental issues. The antimicrobial properties of Goldenseal products help in treating gingivitis and dental plaque. The products kill the bad microbes very easily and also prevent these problems from coming back again.

Likewise, the anti-inflammatory power of the Goldenseal root also takes care of the inflammation in any sore gums. It brings the discomfort down and helps in eating and drinking easily. The Goldenseal root can be used as a mouthwash or a toothpaste daily to promote brilliant oral health and keep such painful and problematic dental problems at bay.

Chapter 4: Rules to Take Goldenseal for Better Health

Now that we are aware of the vast multitude of health benefits that the Goldenseal root has to offer, it is crucial to understand how you must use the products derived from the rhizome. Let us look at the rules to take Goldenseal for better health.

Many forms in which the Goldenseal root is available

Before we talk about the considerations you need to take care of when consuming Goldenseal root products or the interactions it can have with other medications, it is important to understand the many forms it is available in. This helps us in recognizing which form of Goldenseal works best for us and which ones we should avoid. Due to the structural strength of the Goldenseal root, modern pharmaceutical and herbal medicine companies have been able to process the rhizome in multiple forms. It can be dried into a powder or turned into an aqueous concoction. It can also be processed and manufactured as pills or capsules or a tincture that can be applied directly to the skin.

As raw root

The most common form in which the Goldenseal root is available is the raw root form. Even though it is readily available in the market, it is advisable not to consume it raw. One can boil the raw Goldenseal root in water and prepare a solution or steep the raw root in tea as well. We highly recommend doing so in chamomile, sage, or eucalyptus tea. Once the solution is well boiled, one can drink it as it is. This method of Goldenseal intake is simple and efficient. Plus, the entire process doesn't take any longer than fifteen minutes. The Native Americans used this very method popularly and found no issues in this form of consumption. If you boil the Goldenseal root in plain water, you can also use this solution as a wash to clean your eyes.

As a powder

Another popular form in which the Goldenseal root is available in is the powder form. The Goldenseal root is dried and then crushed into a powder form for easy consumption. Most powdered forms of the Goldenseal root have berberine as the major constituent. So, if you find a product with berberine written on it, you know that it was derived from the Goldenseal rhizome. This powder is very versatile to use. You can mix an appropriate amount of it in water and drink it. You can even use this solution to clean wounds or rub it on an infected area. Make sure to clean up with plain water after you have used the Goldenseal solution on any body part. Other than water, one can also mix the powder in fruit juice. This forms a tasty solution which one can then drink easily. You can pair up your juice with any breakfast item or have it as a snack during brunch time as well.

As pills and capsules

These two forms of Goldenseal products are not only commonly available but were also the most famous forms with the Native Americans. It was only after the commercialization of the yellow rhizome that it became available in alternative forms. Pills and capsules are processed forms of the Goldenseal root. Pharmaceutical companies carefully decide upon the concentration of the various chemicals present in the root that need to go into the pill or capsule. Highly toxic chemicals are removed from the product, and only non-toxic chemicals are put in. These pills and capsules can be easily found in pharmacies or local drug stores. It makes it very easy for people to consume them since they do not have to drink a solution or eat it in powder form. This way, you can control the dosage of the root as well.

As a tincture or extract

The Goldenseal root is also available as a tincture or an extract. This is a concentrated solution or a salve-like paste which is usually used directly on the problem area on your skin. These Goldenseal tinctures or extracts are very useful to treat the skin conditions one might have. Since they are directly applied to the problem area, their rate of effectiveness increases tremendously. So, if you are suffering from skin problems like eczema, you can choose to buy a Goldenseal tincture or extract rather than its pills or powder forms. Plus, they can also be used effectively in dealing with hair-related problems. Simply apply the extract on your scalp to deal with dandruff or to get healthier and more luscious hair. Using a Goldenseal tincture can also work as a hair tonic.

In cosmetics and body creams

The anti-inflammatory, antimicrobial, antiseptic, and antioxidant properties of the Goldenseal root are very well known. There's no doubt about the fact that the yellow rhizome is a great supplement to boost hair and skin health. Plus, the Goldenseal root is loaded with vitamins and minerals. This makes it an even healthier choice for both clean skin and lusciously growing hair. The numerous health benefits of the Goldenseal root caught the attention of several cosmetics and personal care brands, and they decided to incorporate its goodness in their products as well. The extracts of the Goldenseal root can now be easily found in over-the-counter cosmetics. Be it facial serums or soothing lotions, the Goldenseal extract helps boost healthy skin.

Berberine is the main component in these products, and it not only helps in getting clean and healthy skin but also to deal with any harsh sun exposure. These personal care products are highly suitable for people who have sensitive skin. The isoquinoline alkaloids help in treating blemished skin and relieve the symptoms of acne, eczema, psoriasis, and more. The Goldenseal root extracts are also available as facial cleansers or after-sun soothing lotions that can softly bring relief to your sensitive skin and also deal with the damage done. Body creams and lotions containing the Goldenseal extract can also provide intense moisturization as well as bring down inflammation, prevent infections, keep the skin squeaky clean, and also provide radiant glow and health.

Dosage, frequency, exceptions related to the consumption of the Goldenseal root

Now that we are aware of all the different types of Goldenseal products available in the market for us, it is also crucial to understand how one should consume it. The correct dosage, the right frequency, and certain precautions are necessary to ensure the consumption of the Goldenseal root causes no side effects. It also helps you make use of the complete potential of the yellow rhizome effectively. Note that, different products come with different dosage recommendations. Your recommended dosage also changes depending upon your age, height, weight, and medical ailment that you are trying to target.

Dosage and frequency

The recommended dosage for dried Goldenseal root consumption is 0.5–10 grams three times a day. If your medical condition isn't very serious or your weight isn't a lot, you will most likely be put on a lower dosage of the Goldenseal root. Likewise, a person with a heavier body weight might be put on a higher dosage. The idea is to ensure that you do not consume way too little or way too much of the rhizome. It is also important to space out the dosage of it over the day. Similarly, if you are looking to try out alcoholic tinctures or aqueous extracts of the Goldenseal root, the recommended dosage is anywhere between 0.3–10 mL thrice daily.

For people who are looking to use the Goldenseal root as an everyday herb, using it in its powder form is the best and easiest way to go. The powder is available in any general or herbal store. You can take about two teaspoons of the

powder and steep it in one cup of hot water to prepare tea.

Fifteen minutes is a good enough time for this. You can then

let the tea cool down for a little bit and consume it.

Depending on your needs, drink this tea two or three times

a day. While there has been no certain evidence regarding

the potential effects of an overdose of the Goldenseal root,

it is advisable not to go above the recommended dosage.

There is a chance that too high a dosage of the rhizome can

result in toxicity; however, this is highly unlikely with

Goldenseal products that have been manufactured by

pharmaceutical companies. In any case, it is important that

you

consult your doctor before consuming the herb and not self-

medicate.

Side effects of the rhizome

Even though there is no evidence of overdose, there are still

a few side effects associated with the wild herb. These side

effects are usually very rare and only occur in a few cases.

Two of these rare side effects include nausea and vomiting. Some people might experience both of them together or individually as well. There are also rare cases where people might experience reduced liver function. However, all of these side effects are very rare. These side effects are also mostly seen in people who consume products that claim to be the Goldenseal root, but the ingredients aren't those of the root. This is why it is crucial for you to carefully read the labels on these products and ensure that it contains ingredients derived from the Goldenseal root and not from its substitutes

like Oregon grape root or Chinese goldthread.
Ensure that the product label mentions the important isoquinoline alkaloids like berberine, hydrastine, canadine, and palmatine. These labels might also mention ingredients like Vitamin A, B, C, and E and other minerals like zinc and iron. Also, look at the concentration of the product and see if it is below or above the recommended levels. If the concentration is not right, the constituents won't be absorbed by the body adequately, thereby resulting in poor

or no results. As a precaution, it is always wise to consult your doctor before starting to consume any product that mentions the Goldenseal root to be an ingredient.

Possible interactions of the Goldenseal root

The yellow rhizome is relatively very safe to consume. There is currently no evidence of overdose resulting from the root or of any severe side effects. However, there is a possible interaction that can affect the root's potency and threaten other body functions. Certain medications, like antidepressants, require timely elimination from the human body. Several liver enzymes are involved in this process, and it is crucial for their production to be timely and in the correct quantity and capacity. In case that the activity of these liver enzymes is slowed down, antidepressants do not get eliminated from the body as they should.

Accumulation of these medicines in the body for long durations can result in high toxicity of the medicine and enhanced side effects. It could also lead to an overdose of the antidepressants. Thus, if you are on any kind of antidepressant, you must refrain from using the Goldenseal root in any form. The wild herb slows down the action of liver enzymes and can result in toxic accumulation of the antidepressants in your body. Other than this, it is also advisable for pregnant women and children not to consume the root in any form. Since berberine has an effect on uterine muscles and causes them to contract, the Goldenseal root can induce preterm labor in pregnant women.

The Goldenseal root can also result in low birth weight of the newborn baby and can also cause jaundice in the babies. If babies or children are already suffering from jaundice, the usage of this herb can worsen the condition. The wild herb also has an effect on the neurons in the brain, and the usage of the same in developing babies and children can result in adverse side effects. Thus, it is advisable for both pregnant women and children not to consume any product derived from the

Goldenseal root. The wild herb has shown no interactions of side effects from breastfeeding mothers to their children. However, due to the lack of any solid evidence, it is recommended for breastfeeding women to avoid its consumption as well. The Goldenseal root is generally considered to be safe for consumption by teenagers and adults.

Usage of the Goldenseal root along with Echinacea

There is always something that enhances the effect of the other. For example, the consumption of Vitamin D enhances the absorption of calcium in our bodies. This makes the effects of calcium supplements very good. Similarly, there are products that enhance the effects of the Goldenseal root as well. One such product is Echinacea. Echinacea is a purple cone-flower, which is a Native American wild herb found mostly in the plain states. This herb has been used as a medicinal plant in American and European communities for over a century. Amongst the many medical benefits that Echinacea offers, a few of them include:

- Reducing the effect of cough, colds, flu, and other bacterial and viral infections of the throat and lungs.
- Treating several poisonous snake bites like rattlesnakes.
- Dealing with pain and inflammation.
- Lowering the intensity of migraines and other such headaches.
- Lowering sugar levels to deal with chronic diseases like Type II Diabetes Mellitus.
- Helping improve immunity levels to make your body healthy.
- Repairing your skin's outer layers to deal with conditions like eczema and skin inflammation.
- Treating urinary tract infections, especially in women.

These are just a few of the health benefits that Echinacea offers and it does not cause any side effects similar to the Goldenseal root. In very rare cases, the oral consumption of the Echinacea root can cause rashes or worsen asthma in patients who are already suffering from it. Other than this, there is no evidence of any side effects caused by Echinacea.

Clearly, it has low toxicity and is highly safe for consumption. Like the Goldenseal root, the Echinacea extract is also available in numerous forms - powdered, liquid, pills, capsules, tinctures, and more. The power of both Echinacea and the Goldenseal root is enhanced in magnitude when both of them are taken together.

Since both Goldenseal and Echinacea are active immune system developers, using them together enhances the effects of each. Plus, both can together help in bringing down inflammation faster. This is exceptionally powerful in bringing down inflammation in patients suffering from neurodegenerative diseases like Alzheimer's, Parkinson's, and other types of Dementia. In patients suffering from these diseases, the brain cells become incredibly inflamed, which worsens its symptoms such as memory loss, reduced coordination, feeling spacey and disoriented, losing cognitive abilities of reasoning, problem-solving, and more. While Echinacea and the Goldenseal root both can bring down the inflammation individually, using them together can be quite the game-changer.

Like the Goldenseal root, one can also take the Echinacea extract as a powder, in tea, as a pill or a capsule, or use it as a tincture or extract to be applied directly on the skin or in your hair. While the recommended dosage remains the same as the Goldenseal root, it is highly advisable that you consult with your doctor before taking the two herbs together. Herbal medicines usually have very low toxicity and are relatively safe to be used in combination than other pharmaceutical drugs. However, like any other medicine, there are a few considerations that you must make before consuming the Goldenseal root and Echinacea in combination.

Please note, pregnant women should steer clear of this herbal medicine unless advised by their doctor. Since the research on the effect of both the Goldenseal root and Echinacea on pregnant women and developing babies is limited, it is highly advised that you do not experiment with the combination. That being said, breastfeeding mothers and toddlers shouldn't be given the Goldenseal root nor Echinacea as well. Again, if you are on antidepressants, consult with your doctor before using this herbal medicine. Other than this, there are no proven interactions shown by both these Native American wild herbs. They both offer very low or non-existent toxicity levels even at high doses and do not have any side effects. This makes this wonder duo not only a powerful remedy for a host of medical ailments and conditions, but also a very safe alternative medicine for patients who do not like to consume traditional forms of pharmaceutical medicines.

Goldenseal root recipes to try out

Even though the Goldenseal root is available for consumption in several forms, some people might still be reluctant to try them out. Some wouldn't want to eat a powder while others wouldn't want to drink a solution. There are also several patients who get extremely reluctant and fidgety when they need to take their medicines. For all such cases and more, we always have the option to use this medicinal herb in a recipe. Additionally, consuming the

Goldenseal root this way also makes it look less like medicine and more as a snack, thus making you feel that you aren't constantly medicating yourself. Let us look at a few of the most amazing recipes that involve using the Goldenseal root.

The Goldenseal root infused Tea

Ingredients

Goldenseal root in powdered form (can be easily found at any pharmacy or herbal store)

2 to 3 cups of water

Raw honey, to taste (optional)

Teabags of your favorite tea, we recommend eucalyptus, chamomile, or sage (optional)

One teaspoon of Echinacea (optional)

Prep time

2 minutes

Cook time

20 minutes

Instructions

In a kettle or a boiling pan, bring 2 to 3 cups of water to a boil. Once the water begins to bubble, simmer down the flame or take the kettle off the flame altogether. In a teacup, add one teaspoon of the Goldenseal root powder. To this cup, gently add the boiling water. At this step, if you'd like, you can also add a teaspoon of the Echinacea extract. This helps you get relief from your symptoms faster. However, consult your doctor before adding this to your recipe. Now, once you have filled the cup with boiling water, let it steep for about 15 to 20 minutes.

Again, before you let it steep, you can consider adding a teabag of your favorite flavor as well. This simply enhances the experience of drinking Goldenseal tea and lets you enjoy it to the fullest. This step is, again, optional. Once you have let the tea steep for about 20 minutes, strain out the powder using a strainer. It is important to do this without fail since you do not want the powder to come in your mouth when enjoying your cup of tea.

Do note that this tea thus steeped can be very bitter. If you are not affected by this, you can have the tea as it is. However, since the entire point of this recipe is to help you elevate the experience of consuming the Goldenseal root, we highly recommend adding something to the tea that can improve its flavor. This can either be done by adding a teabag of your favorite flavor of tea or by adding raw honey to your taste. Ensure that the honey doesn't have any added sugar. This is exceptionally important for people who are consuming the Goldenseal root to relieve symptoms of Type II Diabetes Mellitus.

Since this recipe takes barely any time to prepare and cook, it is one of the most highly recommended recipes involving the Goldenseal root. It is simple and efficient and requires barely any technical cooking skills. However, if you wish to jazz things up a little and elevate your experience further, you can also try our highly recommended recipe for the Elderberry Syrup prepared with Goldenseal and Echinacea. Here, again, the Echinacea extract is optional.

The Elderberry Syrup with Goldenseal and Echinacea

Ingredients

Goldenseal root in powdered form (can be easily found at any pharmacy or herbal store)

3 to 4 cups of water

1 cup of dried Elderberries (can be found at a local grocery store)

A piece of ginger (about two inches in length)

2 sticks of cinnamon

5 to 6 cloves

Raw honey, to taste (optional)

One teaspoon of Echinacea (optional)

Prep time

5 minutes

Cook time

1 hour 30 minutes

Instructions

The instructions for this recipe are quite simple. In a large
pan or pot, add about four cups of water. Put the flame on
high and bring this water to a boil. Next, add all the herbs
and spices (Goldenseal root, elderberries, ginger, cinnamon,
cloves, and Echinacea) into the vessel together. Bring this
mixture to a rolling boil. Once you begin to see bubbles of
water in the pot, simmer down the flame and let the
mixture stay on the heat for the next 45 minutes to an hour.
Stir occasionally to ensure nothing sticks together. Once you
have boiled and reduced the solution for about an hour,
switch off the flame and take the pot off the stove.
Strain out all the berries, herbs, and spices using a strainer.
Now, it is crucial to let this syrup rest for at least half an

hour. Do not consume the syrup straight off the stove since it is very hot. Plus, the current syrup you have is very spicy and strong. Not everyone would be able to tolerate such a strong taste. To cut the strong and spicy taste, we highly recommend adding a dash of local raw honey. The sweet taste of the honey and the added goodness of its health benefits help finish off the recipe superbly. Remember, add honey to taste to the pot only when the syrup has cooled down properly. Adding honey to a hot mixture ruins its health benefits.

The Elderberry syrup - without the Goldenseal root powder and Echinacea extract - has been used for several centuries as a homemade remedy for colds, flu, fever, and more. If you wish, you can consume this syrup twice a week without any issues. However, if the syrup needs to be given to a pregnant woman, breastfeeding woman, infant, or toddler, it is advised not to add either the Goldenseal root or the Echinacea extract. In any other case, this syrup can be consumed as it is without any adverse side effects. Since the

Elderberry syrup is very tasty, anyone can have it without worrying about the bitter taste.

The Goldenseal root and Echinacea Jelly

Ingredients

Goldenseal root in powdered form (can be easily found at any pharmacy or herbal store)

4 envelopes of gelatin (unflavored)

1 cup of water or 1 cup of cold juice of your favorite flavor

Raw honey, to taste (optional)

Teabags of your favorite tea, we recommend eucalyptus, chamomile, or sage (optional)

One teaspoon of Echinacea (optional)

Cinnamon sticks (optional)

Dried ginger root (optional)

Prep time

5 minutes

Cook time

3 hours 30 minutes

Instructions

You can either brew your favorite flavor of Goldenseal tea or use your favorite juice to get started. See "The Goldenseal root infused Tea" recipe to learn how to brew it. You can also use both of these solutions. Our recommended juices to be used for this recipe include orange juice, pomegranate juice, cranberry juice, or guava juice. You can also add a dash of the apple cider vinegar juice if you'd like. Our recommended flavors of tea include sage, eucalyptus, peppermint, or chamomile. In a large pot, add all of these solutions along with the herbs and spices mentioned in the ingredients list above, mix well, and let it come to a boil. After about 15 minutes, take it off the heat and let it cool down a bit.

In another large bowl, add your choice of juice and then place the unflavored gelatin in it. Let this stand for about a minute or so and then gently stir in the previous mixture prepared. Once the gelatin has dissolved completely, stir in a little bit of honey to your taste. Again, use raw and local honey that doesn't contain any added sugar. Now, pour the solution in a large flat pan and refrigerate it for at least three hours. Once the jelly has become firm, take it out of the refrigerator and cut them into pieces of your desired height. You can even use cookie cutters of different shapes to jazz up the appearance of the jelly!

Chapter 5: Conclusion

The Goldenseal has been long used as a potent and effective medicinal herb by Native Americans, Europeans, and many others. It has helped people deal with a host of different health problems. Current pharmaceutical drugs are only able to cater to a set of two or three issues at maximum. A drug that helps with reducing fever will not be able to deal with jaundice or relieve symptoms of Alzheimer's disease. You need a host of different tablets and pills to deal with such a wide range of ailments. However, the Goldenseal root changes all of that very easily. It can help you get relief from cough and cold, reduce inflammation from a skin disorder like eczema, treat a fungal infection, treat a stomach infection, relieve symptoms of numerous types of neurodegenerative diseases, and even treat certain forms of cancer.

The availability of the Goldenseal root in multiple forms - powder, tinctures, extract, pills, capsules, and more - makes it easy for people to consume it in the manner they wish.

Those uncomfortable with popping pills can try the tincture or the powder form while others who do not like eating the powder can even try out different recipes to make consumption of the wild herb easier. The capability of this wild Native American drug is phenomenally powerful and deserves more recognition and wise-scale adoption. It also offers several benefits that has nothing to do with medical ailments. Any form of the Goldenseal root can be used as an everyday herb.

Using it regularly can help you get a glowing and healthy skin. Applying the Goldenseal extract on your scalp can also help you get a clean scalp and lusciously healthy hair. Daily consumption of this herb also enables us to maintain top-notch digestive health and keeps our immunity up against common ailments like seasonal flu and fever. No other known pharmaceutical drug is capable of showing positive effects in such a wide range of medical issues. What makes this wild herb even more interesting is that it has very low toxicity even at high doses. This means that the yellow rhizome won't cause any side effects in patients who require a high dosage of it for prolonged periods.

Clearly, the Goldenseal root is a wonder herb that can help you tackle numerous medical issues with complete ease. You don't have to worry about an overdose, severe side effects, or even inefficiency. It is potent, capable, and highly effective. The numerous tasty recipes available that make use of the Goldenseal root is an added benefit to this rhizome. If you wish to lead a healthy life wherein you don't have to worry about serious medical issues, you must consider trying out the Goldenseal root today. Boost its potency with the Echinacea extract or consume it alone in any form you love and find comfortable. Consulting with your doctor and beginning your day with a fresh cup of the Goldenseal root tea or taking a pill a day might just be the best decision you ever make for your health!

Appendix: References

https://www.christopherhobbs.com/library/articles-on-herbs-and-health/golden-seal-in-early-american-medical-botany/

https://science.jrank.org/pages/3079/Goldenseal.html#:~:text=Native%20Americans%20used%20goldenseal%20as,stimulant%2C%20and%20treatment%20for%20cancer

http://www.mastergardenersmecklenburg.org/goldenseal-hydrastis-canadensis-l-a-long-and-colorful-folk-history-native-plant.html#:~:text=Goldenseal%2C%20a%20native%20plant%20has%20a%20history%20of%20healing.&text=Cherokee%20Indians%20used%20Goldenseal%20root,pneumonia%20and%20several%20digestive%20disorders

https://www.webmd.com/vitamins/ai/ingredientmono-943/goldenseal

https://www.healthline.com/health/goldenseal-cure-for-everything#benefits-uses

https://www.verywellhealth.com/goldenseal-what-should-i-know-about-it-88331

https://www.sciencedirect.com/topics/pharmacology-toxicology-and-pharmaceutical-science/hydrastine

https://www.sciencedirect.com/topics/pharmacology-toxicology-and-pharmaceutical-science/canadine

https://www.sciencedirect.com/topics/pharmacology-toxicology-and-pharmaceutical-science/palmatine

https://www.sigmaaldrich.com/life-science/nutrition-research/learning-center/plant-profiler/hydrastis-canadensis.html

https://www.stylecraze.com/articles/benefits-of-goldenseal-for-skin-hair-and-health/

Goldenseal Tea -

https://www.prohealth.com/library/goldenseal-age-old-

herb-medicinal-potential-80963

Elderberry Syrup with goldenseal and echinacea -

https://www.growforagecookferment.com/elderberry-

syrup-with-echinacea-and-goldenseal/

Goldenseal & echinacea jelly -

https://commonsensehome.com/immune-boosting-herbs-

in-finger-gelatin/

https://www.healthline.com/health/goldenseal-cure-for-

everything#dosage

https://www.healthline.com/health/goldenseal-cure-for-

everything#dosage

https://www.christopherhobbs.com/library/articles-on-

herbs-and-health/echinacea-from-native-american-panceato-modern-phytopharmaceutical/ ,

https://www.christopherhobbs.com/library/articles-on-herbs-and-health/echinacea-and-goldenseal-the-dynamic-duo/

https://www.nccih.nih.gov/health/providers/digest/herb-drug-interactions-science